Calisthenics

30 Bodyweight Exercises for

Beginners

Table of Contents

Calisthenics 1

    An Ultimate Guide for Beginners with 30 Unique Bodyweight Exercises 1

Introduction 4

Chapter 1 – Getting Started 5

Chapter 2 – 30 Unique Bodyweight Exercises 7

Conclusion 36

FREE Bonus Reminder...37

Introduction

How well do you know your body?

Until and unless you won't push your limits, you can't attain productive results regarding your health. This might surprise you, but those who treat their body as a temple and work hard to attain physical and mental peace live a happy, long, and prosperous life.

If you are having issues related to your body weight, then it is high-time you bring a positive change in your life. Just like any other change, this one might also seem a little scary in the beginning, but together we can certainly make it. In order to choose a healthy lifestyle, you need to work on your body.

This is the most important step to attaining an overall balance in your life. Take the first step with us and get yourself familiar with the revolutionary practice of Calisthenics. It is a highly renowned and extremely healthy way to exercise. Calisthenics is considered as an art in itself and consists of various rhythmic body movements that don't require the help of any other apparatus.

One of the best things about Calisthenics is that it can be highly beneficial for weight loss. You can get your body in shape after practicing these amazing bodyweight exercises. In this guide, we have handpicked 30 best exercises for beginners that will provide foolproof results to you.

So what are you waiting for? Are you ready to change your lifestyle?

If your answer is "yes" then buckle up and be ready to shed those extra pounds.

Chapter 1 – Getting Started

Recently, the American Medical Associated has classified obesity as a disease. The stats will certainly surprise you, as over 78 million adults and 12 million kids in America have a serious health condition that is directly related to obesity.

If you understand the gravity of the situation, then you certainly need to take a step right away. Fight against your unwanted body fat that can lead to terrible diseases and might even cause heart failure.

Nobody likes to live a short and troublesome life. If you are reading this guide, then you need to congratulate yourself as you have already taken the first step. You have acknowledged that you need to shed a few unwanted pounds to attain a fit and healthy body.

Now, take the next step and get yourself familiar with these essential calisthenics exercises that will make you accomplish your fitness goal. It doesn't matter how much you weight right now, but after following our expert advice, you can see a radical difference in your body.

All we ask is some time and determination. Calisthenics is an art that consists of various rhythmic movements of our body. By following various sets of exercises that are a part of calisthenics, you can attain a more flexible and fit body.

It is considered as one of the toughest forms of training, as you only use your body weight as a resistance. It features various exercises (like push-ups and sit-ups) that can impart strength to your entire body.

Needless to say, it has plenty of benefits. With calisthenics, you don't have to pay for an expensive gym membership or buy any costly apparatus to reduce weight. It doesn't support any added equipment and provides vital results in less time.

Professionals like Bruce Lee, Mohammad Ali, Jason Statham, and more are considered as proponents of calisthenics. Not only to reduce weight – it can also help you in several other ways as well.

Before we make you familiar with different exercises, let's understand the overall benefit of calisthenics.

1. One of the best things about calisthenics is that you can perform it anywhere you want. It doesn't matter if you are traveling or are out in the woods, you don't have to miss your routine.
2. Compared to weight training, calisthenics is considered pretty easy and won't cause any unwanted injury to your body.
3. It provides speedy results. Since you are resisting your own body, it would lead to neural adaptation and you can see a difference in a few days.
4. Calisthenics doesn't restrain people with respect to their age. It doesn't matter if you are running in your 20s or 60s – you can perform these exercises without any trouble.
5. It can help you accomplish your fitness goal, especially if you are planning to lose some extra pounds.
6. Since it requires a strict training, it will bring discipline in your life. Ideally, you should perform your routine for 6 days a week.
7. Most importantly, it will help you develop your brain and immunity strength. Your reflexes would get better and you would feel "in control" with every passing day.

After all, there is a reason why calisthenics is a part of Special Force's training. It has already changed the lives of millions of people all over the world. It is time you also take this journey and change your life as well.

To make things easier for you, we have handpicked 30 best exercises for beginners in this guide. Warm up a little and move ahead to get it started.

Chapter 2 – 30 Unique Bodyweight Exercises

As stated, calisthenics is all about moving your body in a rhythmic manner. To attain best results, try to move your entire body. There are different kinds of exercises that are specifically targeted to reduce bodyweight. Nevertheless, we will start with the basics.

Always try to come up with a routine rather than performing only a single exercise. In this chapter, we will make you familiar with different routines that can be performed in a set. Before that, let's learn the right way to do different calisthenics exercises.

In order to perform any kind of exercise, you need to make sure that your body is ready. Try to warm up your body before you commence a routine. Running, cycling, stretching, etc. are considered as some amazing ways for warming up your body. You can also experiment a little and perform Zumba or any other activity to warm up your body before starting a routine.

One of the most important benefits of warming up is that it would reduce the occurrence of any unwanted injury. Since after warming up, the oxygen level and overall blood circulation in your body is increased, you can perform various exercises easily. Also, it lubricates your joints, which leads to a better movement of bones.

Additionally, you need to understand that it takes a while to reduce weight in a natural way with calisthenics. Follow a routine for at least a month or two to see a significant difference in your body. Now, let's start with the basics. After performing a warm up for some 10-15 minutes, gradually perform these exercises by taking one step at a time.

1. Forward Lunges

Lunges are probably one of the easiest and safest ways to reduce extra bodyweight from your calves, hamstrings, quadriceps, and core. It improves the health of your spine and can help you develop better coordination of your mind and muscles.

Start from a standing position and let your shoulder blades relax. Keep your back straight and attain a perfect balance.

Now, take forward your right leg and push your body ahead. Make sure that at least 70% of your body weight is on your right foot. Do this, while keeping your back straight.

Go ahead and lower your body a little until your right leg would attain a 90 degree. While doing so, you would realize that your left leg has also attained a 90 degree position.

That's great! You got to hold this position for at least 5 seconds. Even though your left foot would be helping you to balance your body, you need to apply pressure on your right leg to get back again.

After standing up, follow the same process with your left leg and keep it going for at least 10-20 times.

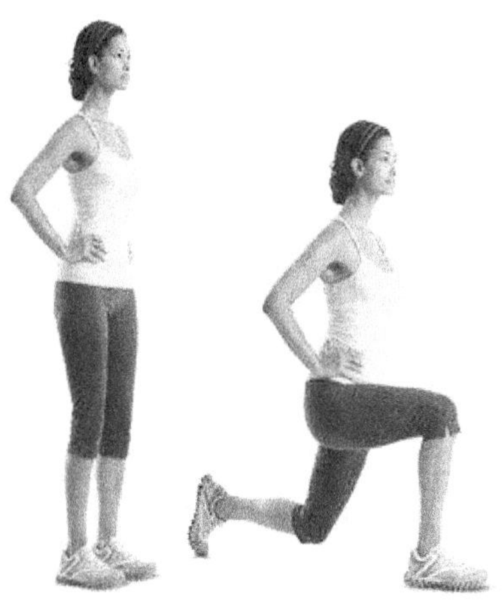

2. Backward Lunges

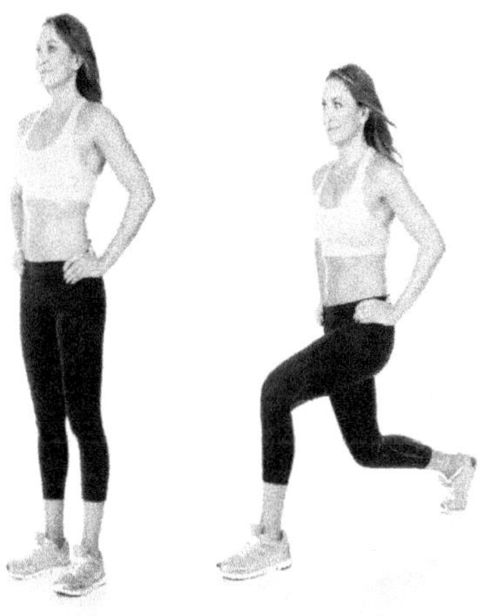

It is just the opposite of the forward lunges. Instead of taking a step forward, start by taking a step back from your left leg and apply the pressure of your body weight towards your back.

Hold this position for a few seconds and use your left leg this time to get back to a standing position. Now, do this with your right leg and keep repeating this rhythm for a while.

Additionally, you can also do the same process sideways by applying alternative pressure to your legs. This is called sideways lunges.

3. Walking Lunges

After mastering forward and backward lunges, step it up a little and try to perform walking lunges. The only difference between forward and walking lunges is that instead of returning back to your initial position, you need to move ahead and walk.

This can be done in a spacious room where you can walk in a circle. Take alternative steps while lunging and performing this productive exercise. Since this would require a perfect balance, it should be done after you have mastered the art of performing regular lunges.

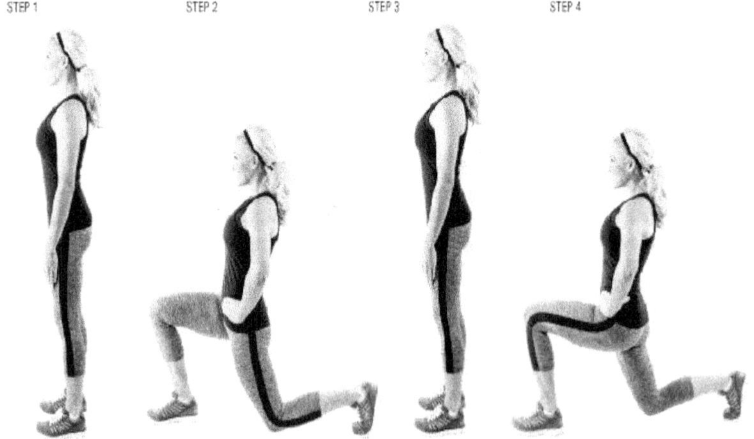

4. Jumping Jacks

This is without a doubt one of the most fun and efficient exercises for beginners. You can do it by putting your favorite tracks in the background as well. After warming up, stand straight and start by bending your knees a little.

Now, propel yourself up and while you are in the air, move your hands as well. You might appear to be in a star-like shape and because of this, the exercise is often known as star jumps.

Move your hands a little as you are going back to the ground and try to cover them behind your head. After heading back on your foot, repeat the steps a few more times. You can easily do it 10-50 times in the beginning.

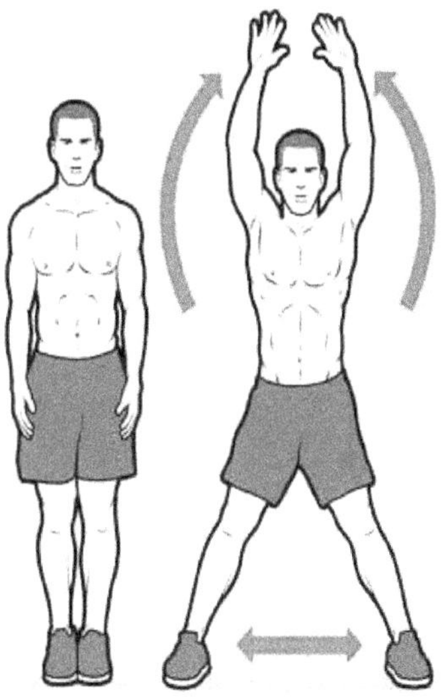

5. Runner Stretch

Stretching is of utmost importance in calisthenics. Not only can it help you warm up but also makes a great routine for beginners. Start by placing your right foot ahead and lower yourself into a lunge position. Now, gradually place your fingertips on the floor. Try to push as much as you can in case you are not able to reach the floor.

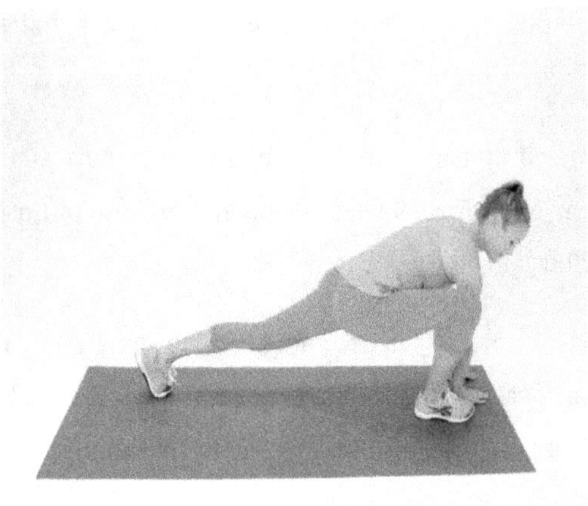

Breathe in and hold this position for a few seconds. Exhale while coming back to the initial lunge position. Switch sides and form a rhythm while doing it at least 5-10 times.

6. Floor Jack Splits

This amazing exercise will help you lose some extra pounds from your frontal area and can develop your abs as well. It is essentially a chest and abs workout. Just lie on the floor to start this exercise.

Put your feet together and unlock your thumbs while stretching your arms and legs. With your own body pressure, lift up your arms and feet at the same time. Make sure that you keep your elbows and knees straight.

Doing this, you would be able to lift your entire body. Now comes the tough part. When you exhale, push a little more and let your arms cross the space between your legs. Slightly reach back to the initial position. Release yourself a little and push back for the next round.

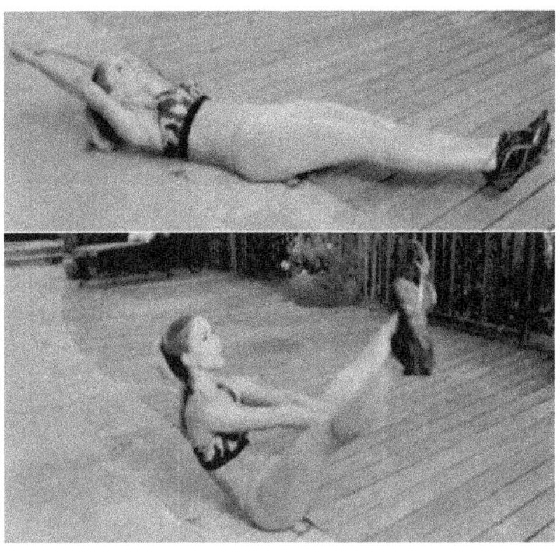

7. Plank Jacks

This would be highly beneficial for your back, quads, arms, and abs. It might be a little hard to do in the beginning, but after a while, you would love the flow.

It is a modified plank position and you need to start by stacking up your shoulders and putting your arms and feet together. When you are in a planked position, keep your body as low as possible.

Now, you need to jump by placing your legs on the opposite sides. Don't stay there for more than a few seconds and jump back to the initial position. Keep doing this for at least 10-50 times.

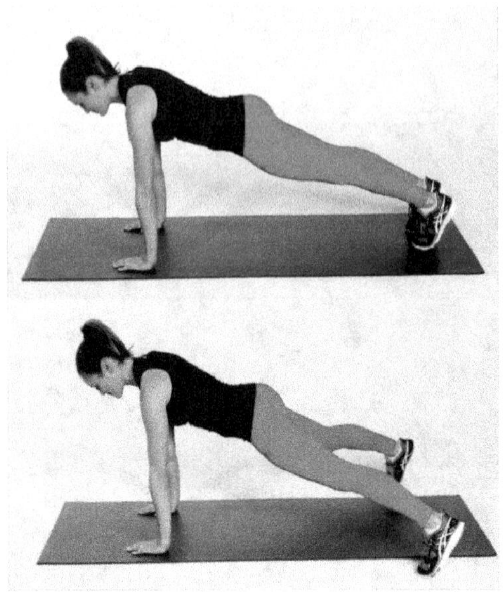

8. Forward Hang

The forward hang is not only a stretching routine, but it can also help you get in shape. The best thing is that it is quite easy to perform. Start this by standing straight. Keep your feet apart and gradually bend your knees. At the same time, interlace your fingers by placing them behind your back.

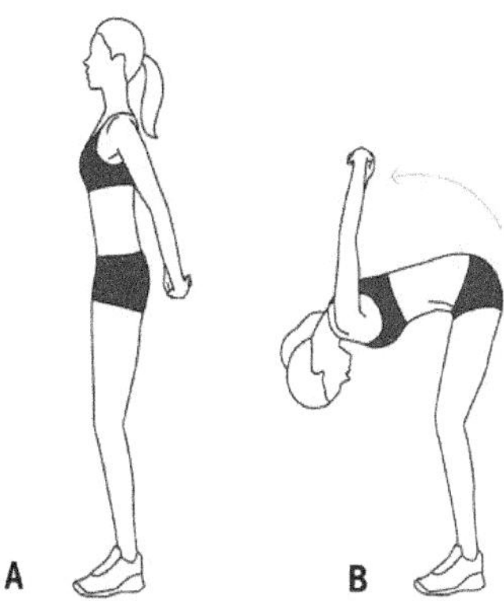

In case your hands are not able to lock, you can hold a cloth or any other lightweight object. Inhale and straighten your arms while expanding your chest. Exhale slowly as you bend your waist. Let your hands stretch upwards and hold this position for a few seconds. Repeat this a few times till you warm up.

9. Squats

Squats are probably the easiest forms of calisthenics. They hold a peculiar importance in any training as they can strengthen your leg muscles and help you reduce weight from your calves.

Start by standing straight and point your toes a little outwards. Now, bend your knees as if you are sitting down. Keep lowering your hips while maintaining your spine in a straight position.

You have to work a little and lower your hips until they would reach the position of your knees. After staying there for a few seconds, you can lift your hips up and come back to the initial position.

Make sure that you keep your spine straight during the entire set. Additionally, you can hold a heavy object (or even a basketball) while doing squats to get better results.

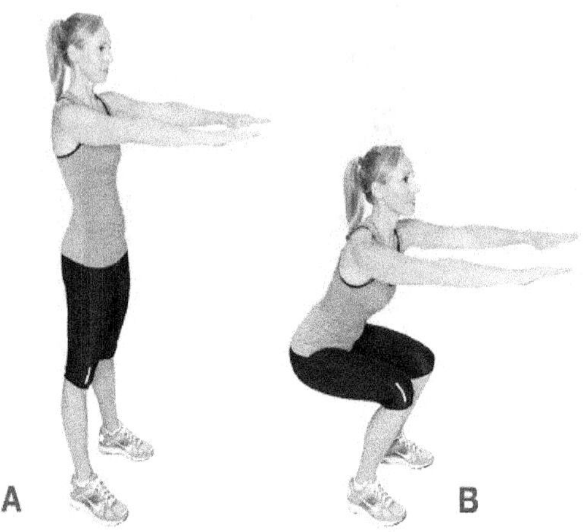

10. Squat Jumps

After performing normal squats, try to level it up and perform a few squat jumps. To perform a squat jump, start by standing straight and initiate by doing a regular squat.

Now, instead of coming back to the initial position, use your body weight and push yourself up a little. Jump up with your core and let go of your hands.

At the time of landing, tactfully lower your body and come back to the initial position as swiftly as possible.

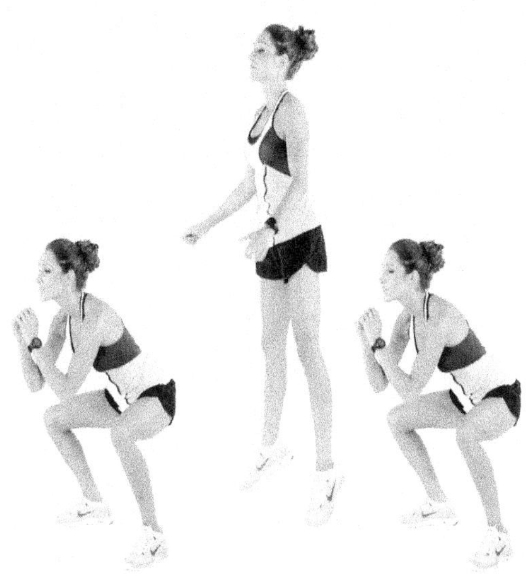

11. Sit-ups

Sit-ups are probably the best ways to provide strength to your abdomen region. Lie down and gradually bend your knees while keeping your foot on the ground.

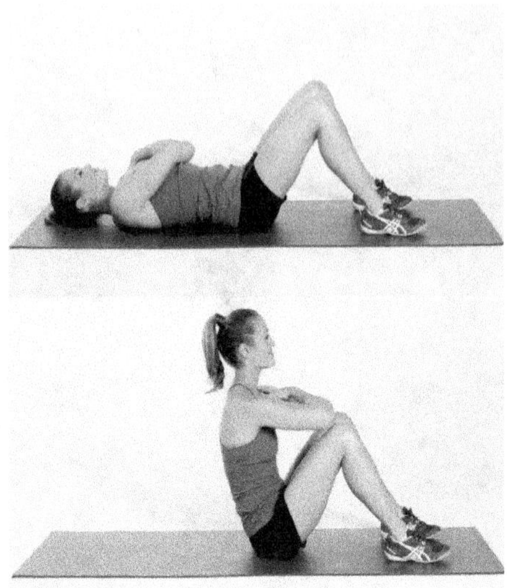

It is also important to cross your arms in order to gain momentum. Tighten your abdomen muscles and gradually lift your head followed by your shoulders. Hold the position for a few seconds and gradually come back to the ground. Repeat this at least 5 times in the beginning.

12. Oblique and bicycle sit-ups

After mastering regular sit-ups, you can always experiment a little and try to perform a different kind of similar exercises.

Oblique sit-ups would be of a great help to you if you are aiming to have abs. When you are lifting your head and shoulders, push a little more and move your body to your either sides.

Similarly, if you like to do the leg work simultaneously, then you can do bicycle sit-ups. When you are performing oblique sit-ups, use your legs and start moving them (as if you are moving a bicycle). When you move your head towards the right side, lift your right leg and subsequently move your left leg when you move your head towards the left side.

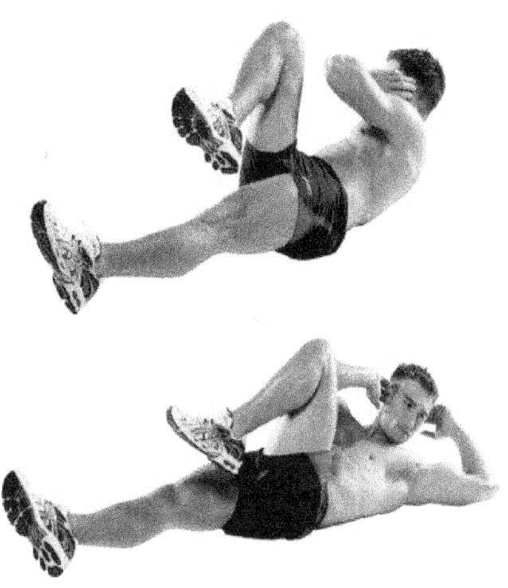

13. Low Lunge Arch

The low lunge arch has a moment, which is similar to yoga. It will help you strengthen your legs and waist. Start by being in a regular lunge position. Now, step your right foot forward and lower your other knee on the floor.

Gradually, bring your arms right in front of your right leg and cross your thumbs together to get some added support. Subsequently, your palms would be placing the floor.

Inhale some fresh oxygen while stretching your arms over your head. Keep stretching them for a few seconds before switching sides. Try to attain a rhythm by doing so 10-15 times.

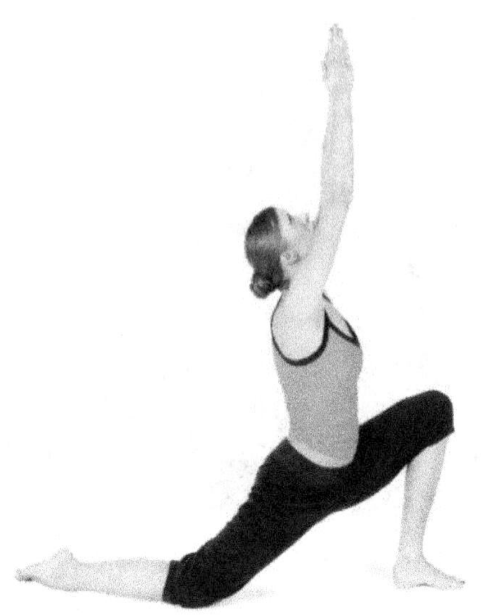

14. Crunches

Just like sit-ups, crunches can also help you shed weight from your abdomen region. If you are able to master sit-ups, then doing crunches won't be that hard for you. Nevertheless, you should pay some extra attention while doing crunches, as most of the people don't know how to do it the right way.

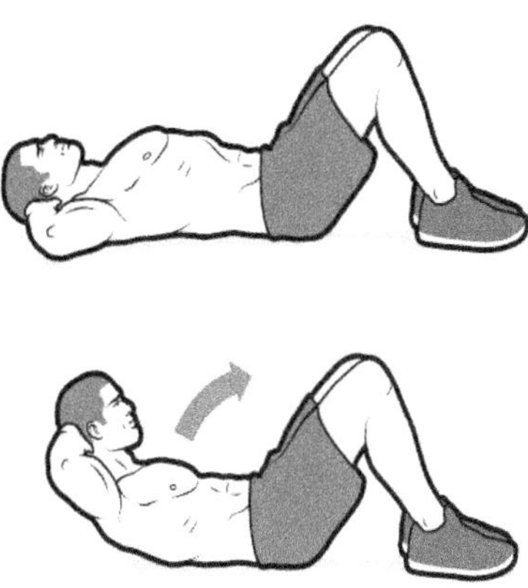

Lie down on your back and bend your knees. Most of the people lace their finger together, which is a mistake. You need to place them behind your head and your thumb right behind your ears (to push your head in the right direction).

Tilt your head slightly and use your body weight and hands to push your head towards your knees. Do this by tightening your abdomen and move forward. Hold still for a moment in that position before going down swiftly.

Additionally, just like sit-ups, there are different kinds of crunches you can practice – like sideways crunches or bicycle crunches.

15. Push-ups

There are different ways to do push-ups. Let's start by understanding how to do a basic push-up. It can radically help you to strengthen your arm and chest muscles.

Start by being in a basic face-down position. Now, you got to raise yourself with your arms. Try not to put pressure on your wrists. There are different kinds of basic push-ups you can do now.

To perform a regular push-up, widen your hands. In order to do a diamond push-up, you need to place your hands together and lay focus on your arms. Simply widen your arms to do a wide-arm push-up. This is done when you need to put focus on your chest instead.

Lower down by choosing the right kind of structure. Don't use the rear end of your stomach while coming down and going back again. Move your chest and lay focus on your arms. Keep doing this for at least 5-10 times in the beginning.

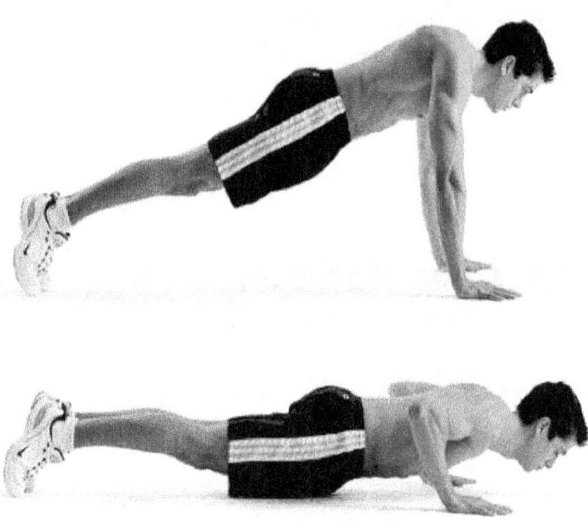

16. Advanced push-ups

There are different kinds of advanced push-ups. The clap push-ups are quite famous though. Start it as a regular push-up and then when you are in the mid-air, clap your hands by applying an extra push.

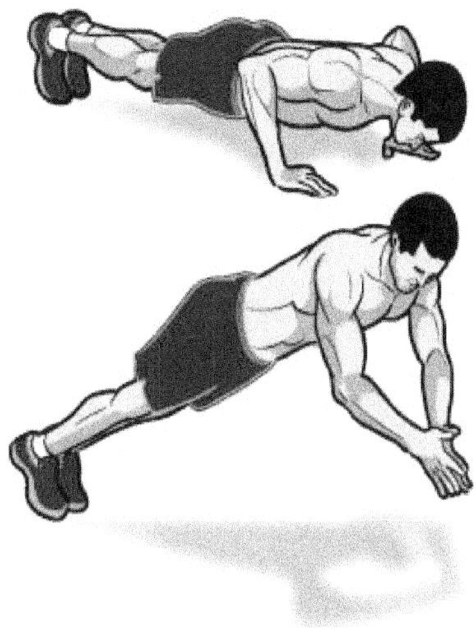

Scorpio push-ups are also quite famous. Start it the same old-fashioned way. Just when you lower your body, raise either left or right leg and bend your knee towards your back. Repeat it by using alternative legs every single time.

There are different kinds of advanced push-ups like one armed, fingertip, knuckle, elevated push-ups, and more.

17. Seated Back Twists

While back twists can help you attain a healthy spine, the seated back twist can boost your overall flexibility as well. Start by simply sitting on the floor (or a mat) and keep your legs straight.

Gradually, bend your right knee and place your foot over your left leg. Keep your right hand on the floor while pointing your fingers outwards. This will support your body posture. Start bending your left elbow and place your arm against your right knee.

Hold this position for a few seconds while inhaling. Now, exhale while twisting a little. Look towards your right while pressing your arm (and not the wrist). Hold again for 10 seconds and gradually come back to the center. You can gradually switch sides and do the same routine with your left leg.

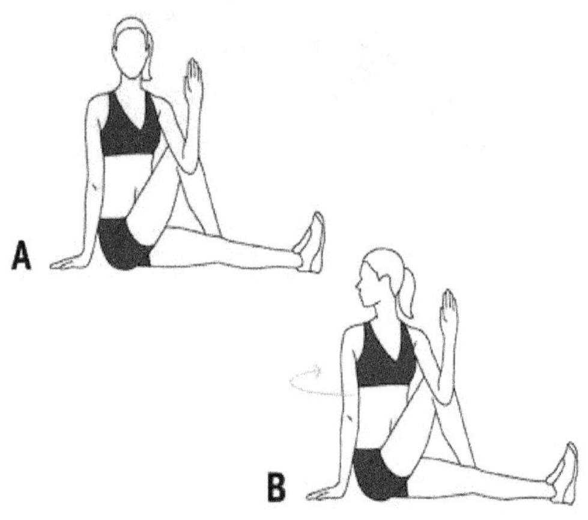

18. Pull-ups

Pull-ups are again a great way to strengthen your upper body, especially your chest, shoulders, and arms. Though, unlike most of the calisthenics routines, you would need a bar to perform pull-ups.

To do a basic pull-up, start by holding a firm grip on the bar. Now, gradually move your body weight using the bar. Try to do this until your chin would come above the bar.

If you are having some trouble, then you can just cross your feet to center your body weight. Gradually lower your body until your arms would be stretched. Do this again for another 5 times to gain momentum.

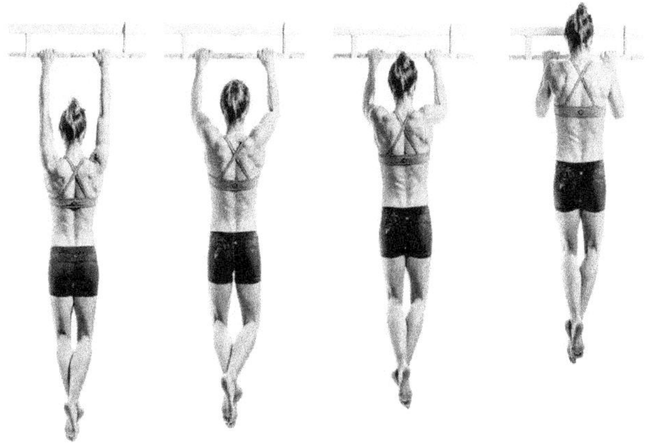

19. Dips

If you can master pull-ups, then you can definitely do some dips as well. You can either get a tool to do dips or even do them with a bench. We will let you know how to do bench dips.

If your bench is not wide enough, then place two of them together. If you are not able to find benches, then you can use a heavy chair as well. Sit down and hold your spine straight while sitting.

Place your palms on the bench and make sure that you have a firm hold on it. Lift your hips and gradually move them down. While doing so, you need to make sure that your spine is straight and that your knees are at 90 degrees.

Try to keep your shoulders relaxed and bend your elbows a little while you lower your body. Using your arms put your body weight back on the bench. Repeat this at least 5 times in the beginning.

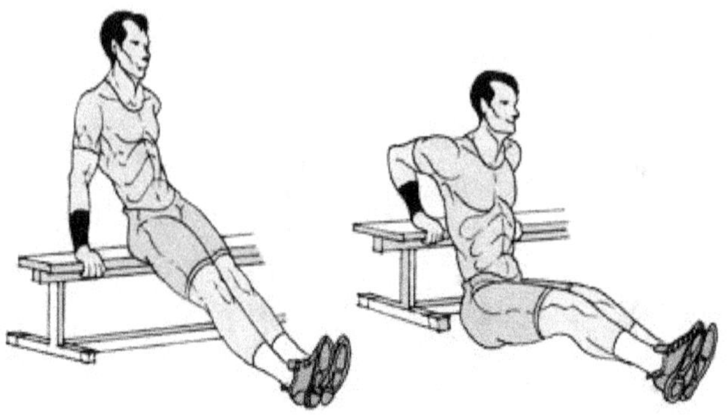

20. Calf Raises

It might surprise you, but you can easily do calf raises without having a machine. They can essentially help you strengthen your calf muscles and lose the extra fat from them as well. Start by holding some heavy object and either face a chair or a wall.

Now, be at least an arm's length distance away from the wall or chair and relax your arms while holding the weight. This is the most important part. Lift your heels up firmly and try to shift the weight on your body with it. Don't bend your legs or spine while doing so.

Stay in that position for a few seconds before lowering your heels. You would feel some kind of a sensation and tension on your calves. Do this for some 10-15 times in the beginning.

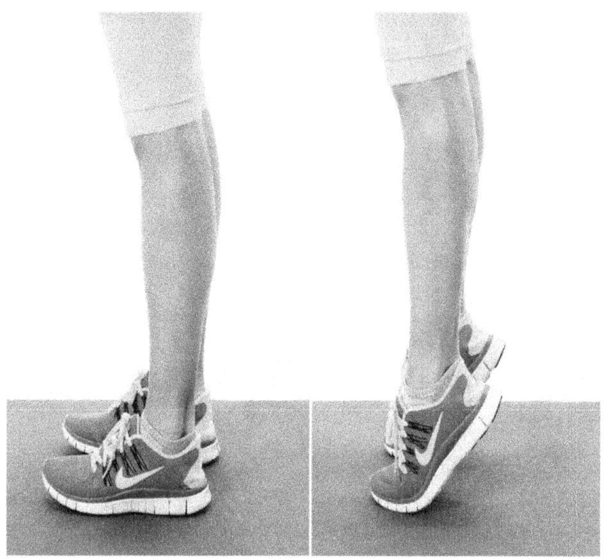

21. Vertical Leg Lifts

If you want to have a great leg work out, then you should definitely give a vertical leg lift a try. Lie on your back to commence this and start bending your knees, gradually to make them at 90 degrees.

Subsequently, move your legs swiftly while keeping your spine straight. Do this until your legs are pointing towards the ceiling. Stay there for a few seconds and then gradually put your legs back to their original position. If you are just starting the set, then prefer doing it at least 5-10 times.

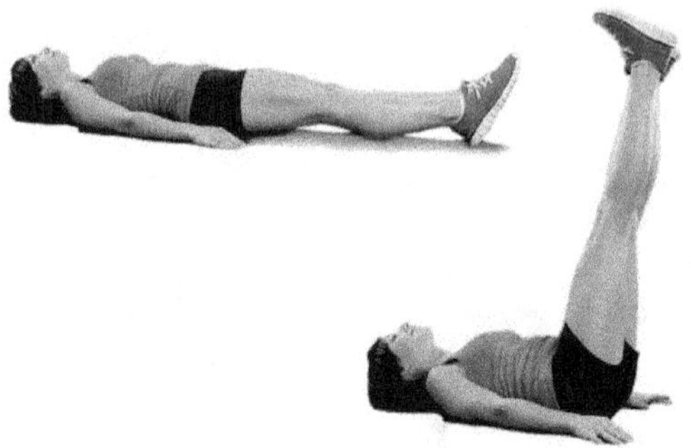

22. Hanging Leg Lifts

After performing some vertical leg lifts, you can change it a little and include a ball between your legs as well. This would make sure that your legs would remain intact and straight while lifting.

There are also different versions of it, including the famous hanging leg lift. After mastering all the basic exercises, you can certainly level it up a little. Include a bar (the one you used while doing pull-ups) and take a firm grip on it. Now, simply hang your body from the bar while holding your arms.

Fold your legs and make them perpendicular to your body. Hold this position for a while and then gradually fold your legs again at 90 degrees. Again, hold the position for another 3-5 seconds and gradually come back to the original state. This will strengthen now only your arms but also your legs and waist.

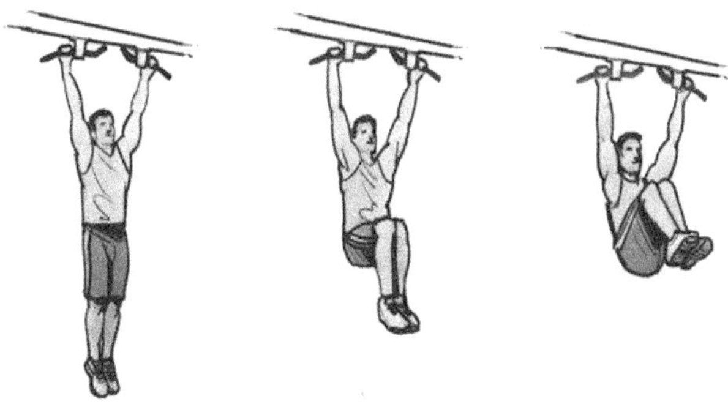

23. Side Leg Lifts

If you think that hanging leg lift is quite tough, then you can try doing side leg lifts as well. This would help you lose weight from your calves. Lie down on one side with your head resting on your folded hands (elbow region).

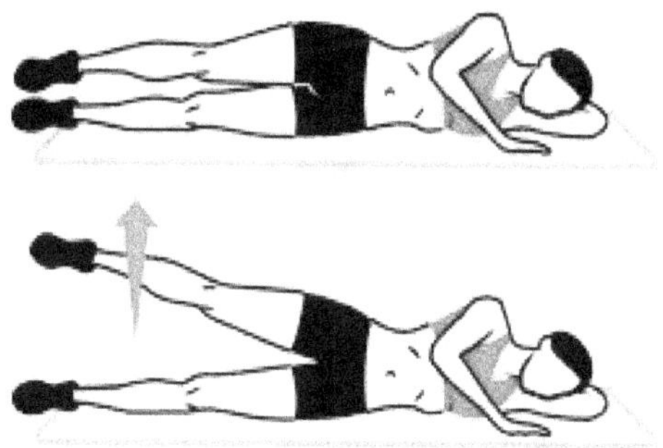

Make sure that you are relaxed before commencing the exercise. Gradually lift your top leg and place it as high as you can. You need to keep your torso and hip region still while doing so. Hold your leg in this position for another 3-5 seconds.

Lastly, lower your leg gently and bring it to its original position. Do it a few times before turning to the other side and doing the same lift with another leg.

24. Bound Angle

The bound angle is an easy and fun calisthenics routine that can help you attain flexibility. Start by sitting comfortably on the floor while keeping your legs straight.

Now, bend your knees slightly and bring your feet together. This would make your knees drop. Hold your legs while inhaling and keeping your spine straight.

Close your eyes for a moment and hold the position. Now, exhale swiftly and hinge forwards by applying body weight. Without turning your back, move your hips forward while placing your hands on the ground. Hold this position for 5-10 seconds before returning to the initial state.

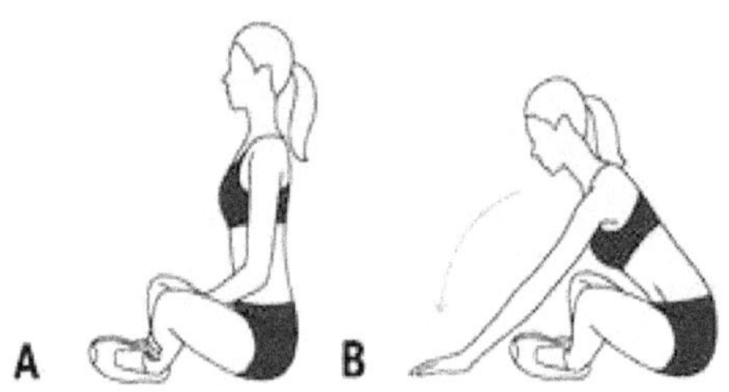

25. Planks

Plank has been originally taken from yoga and has an Indian origin. It is considered as one of the most stringent exercises that can strengthen your core, spine, arms, leg, and shoulders. Let's learn how to do a basic plank first.

Start by being on an all-four position. That is, your knees should be directly beneath your hips and your hands beneath your shoulders. Inhale and exhale gradually now to fill oxygen in your system. Now, start moving your body by making it to a child pose. You need to stretch your hands and breathe by keeping your head underneath. You can even rest your head on the ground or a mat.

After taking five breaths, come forward to a plank pose. Pull long and keep your spine and back elongated. If it becomes tough, then you can even take the support of your forearms and drop down a little. You need to make sure that your stomach is tight at this point.

Hold this position for a few breaths and return back to the child pose while exhaling. This would be counted as one plank.

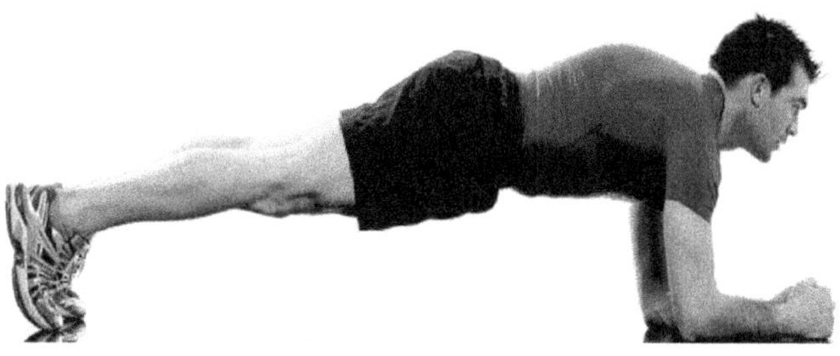

26. Side Planks

These are an advanced form of the regular planks. Start the same way by placing your body in the plank position. Now, instead of simply returning to the child pose, you need to make an effort.

Roll your entire body to the right and let your left hand support it. Stretch your right hand as much as you can and while doing so, make sure that you are resting your weight on your back and arms (and not on the wrist).

After holding for 3-5 breaths, let it go and return back to the plank position. Repeat the process again for the left side before resting.

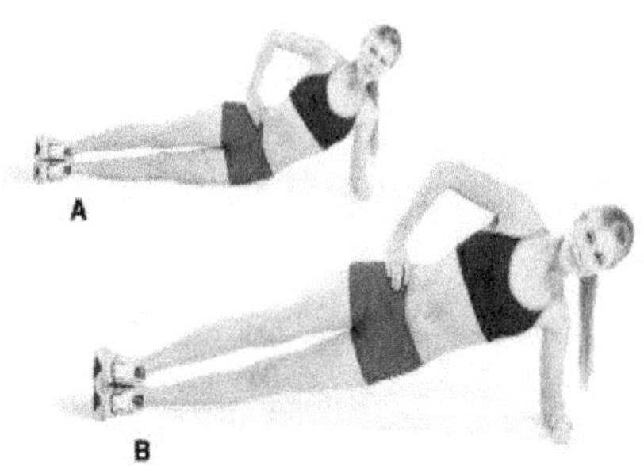

27. Hyperextensions

Hyperextensions are of utmost benefit to your back and spine. Even if you don't have an extension bench, you can use any other kind of support to perform it. Start by resting on the support and make sure that your waist is acting as a fulcrum to move the remaining part of your body.

For the initial position, hold your arms and make sure that your body is in an absolutely straight position. Gradually start by bending your body forward and try to relax your abdomen region. Hold that position for a while before stretching again to the initial position.

You need to ensure that your shoulders are intact and waist flexible while coming back. Repeat this at least 5-10 times in the beginning.

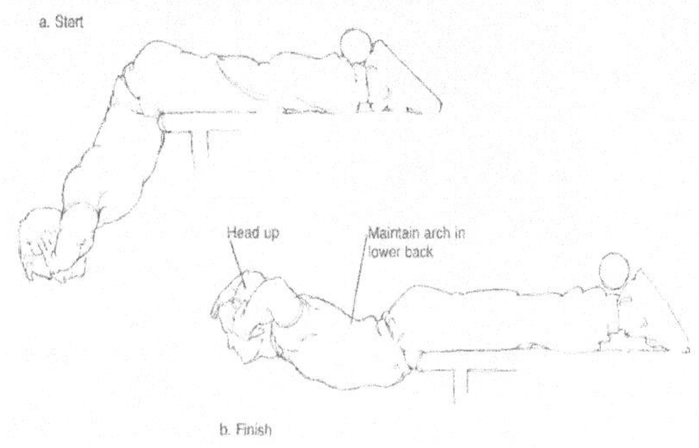

28. Russian twist

Russian twist is an excellent calisthenics workout for those who are trying to lose a few extra pounds from their abdomen and side regions. Start this by sitting on the floor and bend your knees by keeping your feet flat.

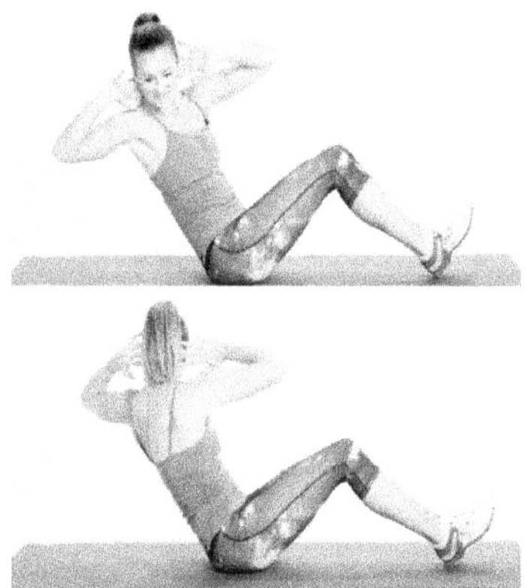

Now, lean back at around 45-degree towards the floor while keeping your spine straight. Keep your arms straight and then gradually lace them in front of your chest. Rotate your core towards the right and hold that position for a while. Do the same movement for the left before returning to the initial position.

29. Frog Hops

Frog hops might seem a little hard to do in the beginning, but they can help you tighten your hip region for sure. The routine is certainly as simple as it sounds. Start by taking the initial plank position. Keep your spine straight and tighten your abs.

Now, with your body weight and using your hips, you need to jump in such a way that your feet would reach your hands. Keep your hands and feet on the floor. You might already feel your lower region getting tighter while bending your spine. Let go and jump again to the plank position. Repeat this at least 10-15 times.

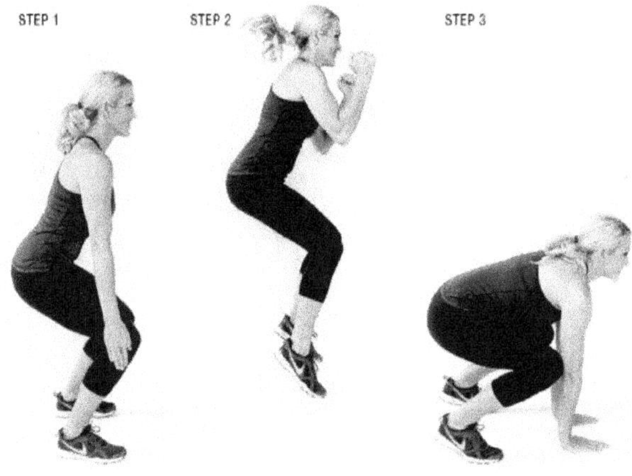

30. Mountain Climbers

The routine is exactly how it sounds. You need to act as if you are climbing a mountain – horizontally. This is an excellent complete body workout that can't be missed.

Start by being in a plank position and tighten your stomach by keeping your spine straight. Now, gradually bring your right knee towards your chest. Here comes the tough part – you can't keep your right toe on the ground. Keep it in the air while putting your weight on your arms and left calves (not on the joints).

Return back to the initial plank position and do the same thing with your left knee. Keep switching the legs until you pick a pace and form a rhythmic pattern.

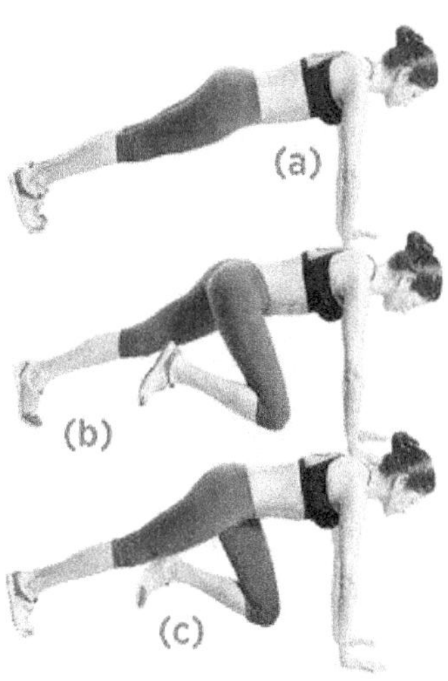

We are sure that after performing these amazing calisthenics workouts, you would be able to bring a major change in your lifestyle. Also, after getting yourself familiar with almost every exercise, try to come up with a routine.

Ideally, a single routine should be of 20-40 minutes and have a mix of various exercises. You can go ahead and create your own routine by including different sets of these exercises. Though, while creating a routine, focus on every part of your body.

Try to attain a diverse routine that would make you focus on your arms, legs, spine, hips, waist, and more. Keep up with your schedule for at least a few months. We sure you would be able to bring a much-needed change in your life.

Conclusion

Congratulations for finishing the book so fast! We are sure you must have had a great time getting yourself familiar with different calisthenics exercises.

No matter how wealthy or successful you are, if you don't have a healthy body and mind then you can't sustain happiness. With the help of various calisthenics techniques that we have mentioned, we are sure you can attain a healthy lifestyle.

To make things easier for you, we have provided 30 different routines that can help you not only to reduce weight but will also strengthen your muscles. Additionally, we have provided an in-depth explanation to perform these routines with their illustrations. We have focused on every part of the body, so that you can have a lean and healthy physique without facing any setback.

So what is stopping you now?

Go ahead and try these amazing sets and come up with a routine for yourself. Don't give up and create a feasible schedule that you can follow. Try to implement your routine without skipping even a single day. With every week, add-on a few sets to make it tougher.

We know it doesn't seem like a piece of cake, but it's not an impossible task as well. In order to achieve greatness, you have to walk an extra mile and give your best. We know you can do this!

www.ingramcontent.com/pod-product-compliance
Lightning Source LLC
Chambersburg PA
CBHW060822260726
48660CB00003B/1055